MOTIVATE YOUR FAMILY TO BE HEALTHIER

A FAMILY GUIDE FOR ALL

CYRIL LAKES

Contents

CHAPTER ONE

INTRODUCTION

It's simple for our health to suffer in today's hectic environment due to our hectic activities. But it's important to put our health first, not only for ourselves but also for our families. Promoting a healthier way of living within your family has several advantages, such as better mood, more energy, and a lower chance of developing chronic illnesses. Even though big changes can seem overwhelming, little measures can lead to long-term enjoyment and health.

We'll look at a variety of tactics and advice in this guide to inspire your family to adopt a healthy lifestyle. We'll examine doable strategies that you can include into your family's everyday routine, from healthy eating habits to consistent exercise and promoting mental well-being. Together, you can motivate your loved ones to take a step toward improved health by creating a supportive environment and setting an example.

Come along as we explore the transforming potential of healthy habits and learn how, little by little, to inspire your family to put their health first.

Family health and well-being are important

It is impossible to overestimate the significance of family health and wellbeing. Families are the foundation of our society, and each member's health and happiness has a significant influence on the strength and contentment of the whole. Family health and well-being should be prioritized for the following main reasons:

Life Quality: Everyone in a healthy family has a higher quality of life. Families can live life to the fullest and participate more completely in activities together when all members are in good physical, mental, and emotional health.

Illness Prevention: Encouraging healthy habits among family members can aid in delaying the start of a number of ailments and long-term diseases. The risk of diseases like obesity, diabetes, heart disease, and some malignancies is decreased by regular exercise, a healthy diet, and preventive healthcare practices.

Emotional Support: During trying times, families are there for each other emotionally. Family members who put mental health first foster a supportive atmosphere where people feel free to express their feelings, ask for assistance when they need it, and manage stress better.

Positive Role Modeling: Children's main role models are their parents and other caregivers. Parents who put their own health and wellbeing first provide a good example that kids are likely to follow. This creates behaviors that last a lifetime and improve long-term health.

Improved Relationships: Family ties are strengthened when members partake in activities that support health and wellbeing, such working out together or cooking wholesome meals. Experiences shared with others generate enduring memories and strengthen a bond and feeling of community.

Better Academic and Work Performance: Cognitive function and academic or professional performance are strongly correlated with good health. Family members are more likely to succeed in their academic and professional efforts when they are emotionally stable, physically fit, and well-rested.

Longevity: A family's adoption of healthy lifestyle practices enhances life expectancy and overall quality of life. Every family member can have a more active and satisfying future by making an investment in their health now.

In order to raise contented, resilient, and successful adults, family health and well-being are crucial. As a family, you may improve the lives of individual members and fortify the basis of your family by placing a high priority on health.

Techniques for Encouraging Family Members

Encouraging family members to put their health and well-being first demands a multidimensional strategy that takes into account the requirements, preferences, and obstacles of each individual.

The following are some methods to motivate and inspire your family members to start living better lifestyles:

Set an example for your family by being the change you wish to see in them. Exhibit healthy behaviors including consistent exercise, a well-balanced diet, stress reduction, and enough sleep. Your family is more likely to prioritize your health if they witness you doing so.

Set Achievable Health Goals: Collaborate with your family members to establish realistic health goals. Whether it's upping daily steps, adding more veggies to meals, or drinking more water, establishing attainable goals can boost motivation and give a sense of success.

Make it Fun: Identify pleasurable pursuits that advance the health and happiness of the entire family. These may be activities like riding, hiking, dancing, sports, or cooking together. Healthy behaviors are more likely to become engrained in your family's routine when they are pleasurable.

Include Everyone: Promote the active involvement of all family members in the decision-making processes pertaining to actions and options connected to health. People are more likely to be involved in the results when they feel heard and included.

Establish a Supportive Environment: Encourage a setting where making healthy decisions is the standard. Provide a healthy food selection for your family, restrict the availability of unhealthy drinks and sugary snacks, and promote candid conversation about health-related issues.

Celebrate Your Successes: No matter how tiny, acknowledge and honor your accomplishments. Healthy behaviors can be strengthened and family members can be inspired to keep moving closer to their objectives by receiving positive reinforcement.

Educate: Share knowledge about the advantages of leading a healthy lifestyle and the negative effects of harmful habits. Give your family the information they need to make wise decisions by educating them on stress management, physical activity, diet, and mental health.

Promote Accountability: Be helpful and nonjudgmental when holding one another accountable. To keep track of objectives and recognize accomplishments, think about establishing routine check-ins or charting progress collaboratively via apps or charts.

Be Adaptable: Recognize that change requires time and that obstacles are an inevitable part of the journey. Be flexible and patient, and be prepared to modify objectives and tactics to take into account personal preferences and obstacles.

Seek Professional assistance: For individualized counsel and assistance catered to your family's unique requirements and circumstances, consult healthcare specialists, nutritionists, or fitness experts as needed.

With persistence, empathy, and patience, you can put these strategies into practice and foster a nurturing environment where family members are inspired to put their long-term health and well-being first.

Probably the most effective way to encourage family members to put their health and well-being first is to set a good example. You provide a powerful example for your family to follow when you exhibit the attitudes and routines you want them to adopt. Here's how to set a good example for others:

Develop Healthy Habits: Integrate wholesome decisions into your everyday activities. This entails consuming wholesome meals, exercising frequently, obtaining adequate rest, properly handling stress, and abstaining from dangerous drugs like tobacco and excessive alcohol.

Be Consistent: Setting a good example requires consistency. Show that you are committed to leading a healthy lifestyle on a regular basis rather than just occasionally. Your family will see how committed you are, and they will be more likely to model themselves after you.

Include Family: Whenever you can, include your family in your healthy routines. Ask them to go on bike rides, hikes, or cook healthy meals with you. This promotes quality family time while simultaneously reiterating how important health is.

Open Communication: Tell your family about your experiences and motivations. Tell them why maintaining your health is important to you and how it makes your life better. Promote candid conversation on health-related issues and show an open mind to their ideas and worries.

Be Resilient: Admit that obstacles are common and that leading a healthy lifestyle isn't always simple. But show resilience by overcoming setbacks and keeping your health as your first priority in spite of them.

Show Balance: Make an effort to maintain equilibrium in all spheres of your life, such as your career, relationships with family and friends, and leisure activities. Prove to your loved ones that maintaining your health improves your general well-being rather than requiring you to give up on other significant elements of your life.

Make self-care a priority. Self-care activities help you to refuel your body, mind, and soul. Set an example for your family by taking time for hobbies, engaging in mindfulness exercises, or making regular doctor's appointments.

Be Supportive and Patient: As you work with your family to develop healthy habits, remember that change takes time. Show yourself and them some patience. Celebrate little accomplishments along the road and provide understanding, support, and encouragement to others.

Lead with Positivity: Take a cheerful and enthusiastic approach to health and well-being. Place more emphasis on the joys and advantages of leading a healthy lifestyle than just limiting or restricting yourself.

Always Learn and Develop: Keep up with the latest findings, developments, and industry standards in the field of health. In order to better promote the well-being of your family, be willing to acquire new techniques and modify your strategy as necessary.

You may set an example for your family and motivate them to prioritize their health and well-being for the rest of their lives by continuously modeling healthy habits and behaviors and fostering an environment that allows them to flourish.

Clearly define your aims and objectives

Setting specific goals and objectives is crucial to inspiring family members to put their health and wellbeing first. While objectives divide more ambitious goals into more manageable steps, clear goals offer focus, direction, and drive. Here's how to help your family set specific goals and objectives:

Determine What Needs to Be Improved: To begin, evaluate the health practices now followed by your family and note any areas that may be improved.

CHAPTER TWO

This could apply to any element of health and wellbeing, including screen time, stress management, physical activity, sleep, and diet.

Establish precise Objectives: For every area that has been identified for improvement, establish precise, measurable, attainable, relevant, and time-bound (SMART) objectives. Instead of aiming for a general objective such as "eat healthier," try establishing a more targeted one like "eat at least five servings of fruits and vegetables per day."

Include the Entire Family: To make sure that everyone feels involved in the process, solicit feedback from each member of the family while establishing goals. Talk about the significance of each objective and how it contributes to the family's overall well-being.

Set Prioritization for Your Goals: Ascertain which of your family's goals are most essential, then order them appropriately. Concentrate on one or two important areas at a time to reduce overwhelm and boost chances of success.

Divide Goals into Objectives: Divide each goal into more manageable, achievable targets that specify the actions required to reach them. These goals ought to be precise, quantifiable, and time-bound so that they may be used as benchmarks to track development.

Create a Schedule: Decide on a deadline for accomplishing each goal and the corresponding objectives. Be realistic about the amount of time needed to make significant changes and take into account both short- and long-term schedules.

Make a Plan: Come up with a comprehensive plan that outlines the tactics and steps needed to accomplish each goal. To facilitate the plan's execution, assign roles, set up procedures, and allot funds as necessary.

Track Progress: Keep tabs on each goal's and objective's advancement on a regular basis to assess success and spot potential problem areas. Maintain family engagement by using tools like apps, notebooks, or visual trackers to show progress.

Celebrate Milestones: To keep momentum and drive going, acknowledge and celebrate your accomplishments at each stage of the journey. Acknowledge both individual and group efforts as well as the strides made toward each objective.

Review and Modify as Needed: Review your family's goals and objectives on a regular basis to gauge progress, spot obstacles, and make any required modifications. Be adaptable and ready to change your plan in response to criticism and evolving conditions.

You may make a successful plan and encourage your family members to put their health and well-being first by setting specific, attainable goals and objectives that are meaningful and catered to your family's requirements.

Encourage Honest Communication

Creating an environment of open communication within your family is essential to inspiring members to put their health and wellbeing first. A friendly environment where everyone feels heard and respected is created through effective communication, which enables the sharing of ideas, concerns, and support. The following are some methods to encourage candid dialogue:

Establish a Safe Space: Provide a trusting and accepting environment where family members may express themselves without worrying about being judged or criticized. Respecting one another's various viewpoints and actively listening to one another will promote open communication.

Set Aside Dedicated Time: Arrange frequent family get-togethers or check-ins to talk about health-related issues, objectives, and worries. Setting aside time for communication allows everyone to participate and demonstrates your commitment to your family's welfare.

Set an example for others to follow by acting with integrity, openness, and respect when interacting with family members. Actively listen to others, respect their viewpoints, and encourage honest communication of feelings and ideas from all.

Encourage Involvement: Motivate every member of the family to take part in conversations and decision-making processes pertaining to their health and wellbeing. Respect everyone's views and make an effort to find out what they have to say.

Pose Open-Ended Questions: To promote meaningful dialogue and in-depth topic exploration, pose open-ended questions. Ask questions like "What are your thoughts on...?" or "How do you feel about...?" to elicit meaningful answers rather than ones that are binary.

Be Empathetic: Be understanding and empathetic with the struggles, emotions, and experiences of family members. Recognize their emotions and, if required, provide assistance and motivation.

Family bonds are strengthened and connected via empathy.

Practice Active Listening: To practice active listening, focus entirely on the speaker, keep eye contact, and try not to interrupt. To make sure you comprehend and to demonstrate your appreciation for their viewpoint, consider back what you've heard.

Constructive Conflict Resolution: Handle disputes or conflicts in a courteous and productive way. Promote honest communication, flexibility, and approaches to problem-solving that put the welfare of the family as a whole first.

Celebrate Progress and Achievements: As a family, commemorate victories and significant anniversaries. Recognize and appreciate any and all efforts made to enhance one's health and well-being in order to encourage positive behavior and keep moving forward.

Seek Professional Help if Needed: If there are underlying problems affecting family relations or if communication hurdles are persistent, you might want to think about getting help from a family therapist or counselor. Stronger family bonds and improved communication can be achieved with the assistance of a professional counselor.

You may establish a supportive environment where everyone feels empowered to prioritize their health and well-being by encouraging open communication within your family. The foundation for cooperation, comprehension, and group development toward a better lifestyle is laid by effective communication.

Make Maintaining Your Health Pleasurable

One important tactic for encouraging family members to prioritize their well-being is to make health joyful and exciting. Engaging and fun healthy activities help them become more sustainable habits that the entire family may enjoy. Here are some suggestions for entertaining your family with health:

Plan family vacations to parks, beaches, or hiking trails so you can all participate in outdoor activities. Explore Outdoor Activities. Engaging in outdoor activities such as hiking, riding, swimming, or playing games outdoors not only encourages physical activity but also offers family time and discovery opportunities.

Turn Exercise into a Game: You may make exercising enjoyable by making it into a challenge or game. Arrange family sports competitions, throw dance parties in the living room, or construct obstacle courses in the backyard. To make physical activity more enjoyable, use apps like fitness trackers to monitor your progress as a team.

Try New Sports or Activities: Inspire family members to participate in new, intriguing sports or pastimes. Taking up new sports, like rock climbing, yoga, martial arts, or dancing lessons, can add excitement and keep things interesting.

Cook Together: Plan and prepare meals with the entire family. Try out new recipes, hold culinary contests, or organize dinner parties with a theme. Inspire innovation and experimentation in the kitchen while imparting useful culinary skills and encouraging a healthy diet.

Plant a Family Garden: Establish a garden that the whole family can help tend to, so that everyone can help plant, water, and harvest fruits, vegetables, and herbs. Growing a garden not only yields fresh vegetables but also strengthens one's bond with the natural world, encourages exercise, and reduces stress.

Host Healthful Potlucks and Picnics: Plan potlucks or picnics where family members bring a dish to share that is healthful. Try out various cuisines and inspire everyone to come up with inventive creations. Family relationships are strengthened and healthy eating practices are reinforced when meals are shared together.

Make Hydration Fun: Add taste to water by adding fruits, herbs, or cucumbers. This will encourage people to drink more of it. Give each member of the family a bright, reusable water bottle and set a challenge for them to drink enough water during the day. Make a hydration game or chart to monitor water intake and encourage it.

Establish Family Challenges: Organize family contests or challenges that center on wellbeing and health. Step challenges, mindfulness challenges, and screen time reduction challenges are a few examples of this. In order to keep everyone engaged, provide prizes or incentives for involvement and accomplishment.

Embrace Technology: Make health engaging and enjoyable by utilizing technology. Look at virtual reality games, online workout videos, and fitness applications that promote exercise. Make challenges or family accounts on fitness apps so you can monitor one other's progress and compete as a team.

Honor Achievements: As a family, honor significant anniversaries and accomplishments.

Recognize and congratulate each family member's accomplishments, whether they are attempting new hobbies, achieving fitness goals, or choosing healthier foods. Healthy behaviors are reinforced via positive reinforcement, which also motivates people to keep participating.

A lifelong good attitude toward health and well-being can be fostered by include delightful and fun activities in your family's routine. In order to keep your family interested and motivated, don't forget to customize activities to their tastes and areas of interest.

Establish a Helpful Environment

Fostering a supportive atmosphere is essential to inspiring family members to put their health and wellbeing first. A supportive atmosphere gives people the tools, skills, and support they need to maintain healthy behaviors and achieve positive changes. Here are some ideas for providing your family with a nurturing environment:

Set a good example for your family members by modeling healthy habits and behaviors yourself. Because you demonstrate by your actions that you value your health above all else, they will be motivated to follow suit.

Promote Open Communication: Create an atmosphere where family members can freely and judgment-free discuss health-related issues. Promote attentive listening and acknowledge each other's worries and experiences.

Establish Realistic Expectations: Steer clear of enforcing stringent regulations or placing unreasonable demands that could make someone feel inadequate or unsuccessful. Instead, appreciate little triumphs along the road and place more emphasis on progress than perfection.

Provide Education and Resources: Make health and well-being-related resources, information, and educational materials accessible. Books, articles, websites, and community initiatives that support healthy living could fall under this category.

Establish Healthy Routines: Make plans and schedules that put the family's overall health and wellbeing first. Allocate specific time for exercise, cooking, resting, and spending time with your family.

Encourage Good Eating Practices: Provide a wholesome food and snack selection for your home, and get the family involved in meal planning and preparation. Promote well-balanced meals and instill in kids the value of choosing wholesome foods.

Make Physical Activity Fun: Look for entertaining methods to include exercise in your family's daily routine. Whether it's walking, playing sports, or dancing to music, make working out a joyful experience for all.

Celebrate Successes: As a family, commemorate accomplishments and significant anniversaries in the areas of health and wellbeing. Recognize and celebrate one another's accomplishments, whether they involve attempting new things, achieving physical objectives, or adopting healthier lifestyle choices.

Offer Support and Encouragement: As family members strive toward their health objectives, offer them support and encouragement. Remind each other that development takes time and work, and provide each other encouragement, support, and advice as needed.

Be Adaptive and Flexible: Be mindful that each person's path to health and happiness is different, and adjust your strategy accordingly. Be open to adjusting routines or tactics as needed to accommodate shifting conditions and personal demands.

Your family can make positive changes and live happier, healthier lives together if you provide a nurturing and supportive environment that supports health and well-being.

Enlighten and educate

To enable your family to make wise decisions and develop healthy habits, it is imperative that you educate and teach them about health and well-being. The following are some methods for enlightening and teaching your family:

Start with the Fundamentals: Provide a summary of the key information regarding the value of health and wellbeing at the outset. Describe the relationship between long life and high quality of life, as well as general physical, mental, and emotional well-being, and healthy practices.

Use Age-Appropriate Resources: Adjust your strategy according to each family member's age and comprehension ability. To communicate important health concepts in an approachable and engaging way, use age-appropriate novels, movies, articles, and internet resources.

Promote Curiosity and questioning: Establish a culture that values curiosity and promotes questioning. Be willing to talk with family members about any health-related issues or worries they may have, and be prepared to answer their questions with factual, evidence-based information.

Give Useful Advice and ways: Give useful advice and ways for implementing healthier lifestyle choices on a daily basis. This could involve advice on hygiene, stress management, sleep, exercise, and nutrition, among other things. Divide difficult ideas into manageable steps that are simple to comprehend and put into practice.

Lead by Example: Set a good example for your family by engaging in healthful activities yourself. Since your behavior speaks louder than words, model good habits by eating a balanced diet, getting regular exercise, learning how to handle stress, and placing a high priority on self-care.

Encourage Critical Thinking: Teach family members to critically assess health information in order to foster critical thinking abilities. Assist them in differentiating between trustworthy and false information so they can make wise decisions regarding their health.

Take Part in Interactive Learning: Make studying health and wellness enjoyable and interactive. Plan family activities such as games, quizzes, experiments, or debates to help reinforce important ideas and encourage involvement.

Keep Up: Remain current on health research, trends, and best practices so that you can give your family accurate and up-to-date information. Adhere to reliable sources, including academic institutions, professional associations, and government health bodies.

Promote Lifelong Learning: Create a culture in your family where people value lifelong learning by stressing the value of always seeking out new information about health and wellbeing. Family members should be inspired to learn new things, pose inquiries, and maintain a healthy sense of curiosity.

Be Patient and Helpful: Acknowledge that gaining knowledge about health is a continuous process. Show your family members your support as they go through their own personal health journeys. Along the process, celebrate their accomplishments, give them support, and acknowledge their hard work.

You may provide your family with the information and tools they need to make wise decisions and live better lives by educating and informing them about health and well-being in a way that is encouraging and empowering.

Assist Everyone in Making Decisions

Including all members of the family in health and well-being decision-making processes promotes a sense of empowerment, accountability, and ownership. The following are some effective ways to include everyone in decision-making:

Have Family Meetings: Arrange for frequent family get-togethers where all members can take part in conversations regarding health-related subjects. Setting objectives, organizing meals, scheduling exercise, and talking about worries and difficulties are a few examples of this.

Establish a Safe Space: Provide a setting where members of the family can freely express their ideas and preferences without worrying about criticism or condemnation. Promote candid dialogue and attentive hearing to guarantee that every individual's viewpoint is acknowledged and valued.

Establish objectives and Goals: To keep conversations focused and fruitful, set objectives for family sessions. Every meeting should have clear goals and objectives. Family members should be encouraged to add issues to the agenda depending on their interests and concerns.

Collaborate to Come Up with Solutions: When faced with decisions or issues pertaining to health, get everyone involved in coming up with possible solutions. Promote innovation and teamwork, and take into account all viewpoints when coming to a decision as a family.

Promote Consensus Building: When making decisions that have an impact on the entire family, try to come to an agreement or make a compromise. Promote polite discussion and debate, and collaborate to develop solutions that take into account the needs and desires of all parties.

CHAPTER THREE

Assign obligations: Depending on the interests, abilities, and availability of each family member, assign tasks and obligations pertaining to health and well-being. Everyone will feel more invested in the results and that tasks are assigned equitably if they are included in the decision-making process.

Individual Preferences Should Be Considered: When deciding on activities or choices connected to health, individual preferences and priorities should be taken into consideration. Acknowledge that every member of the family might have distinct wants and preferences, and make an effort to discover solutions that work for everyone.

Ask Kids for Input: Considering their age, maturity level, and skills, involve kids in decision-making processes for their own health and well-being. Give them the freedom to choose and to voice their preferences within reasonable bounds.

Set a good example for the family by demonstrating courteous dialogue and cooperative decision-making. Demonstrate your openness to hear other people out, take into account their viewpoints, and collaborate to achieve shared objectives.

Evaluate and Adjust: Regularly assess the success of your decision-making procedures and make necessary adjustments in response to input and results. Be adaptable and open to change your strategy to better suit your family's demands.

Involving all members of the family in health and well-being decision-making processes helps foster a sense of cohesion, shared accountability, and support for one another. Collaboration and involvement are encouraged because they guarantee that choices are made with everyone's best interests in mind, which produces more significant and long-lasting results.

Establish wholesome routines and habits

Establishing routines and good behaviors is crucial to building a foundation of health within your family. Regular routines and habits offer opportunity for daily practice of healthy behaviors as well as structure and stability. Here's how to establish routines and good habits that your family can follow:

Establish Priorities: Choose the aspects of your family's health and wellbeing that should receive the greatest attention. This could involve stress management, screen time management, sleep, physical activity, and diet.

Set Achievable and Measurable Goals: For every area of focus, set realistic goals that can be measured. Make sure your objectives are clear, doable, and in line with your family's requirements and preferences.

Establish a Schedule: Make a daily or weekly plan that includes time set out for activities and behaviors that promote health. Set aside specified periods for rest, exercise, eating, sleeping, and other important activities.

Establish Mealtime Routines: To guarantee that nutrient-dense options are always available, plan and prepare balanced meals and snacks in advance. Establish regular meal times and make every effort to eat as a family.

Make Physical Activity a Priority: Set aside time each day for physical activity, such as walking, playing sports, or engaging in active hobbies. For youngsters, try to get in at least 60 minutes of moderate to intense exercise per week, and for adults, aim for 150 minutes.

Make sleep a priority by establishing regular nighttime routines for the entire family to encourage restful sleep. Reduce the amount of time spent on screens before bed, and keep the lighting and temperature at a suitable level to create a peaceful and restful sleeping environment.

Limit Screen Time: Establish limits on the amount of time spent on screens for entertainment purposes, including TV, video games, and social media. Promote substitute activities that enhance social connection, creativity, and physical activity.

Maintain Good Hygiene: Stress the value of maintaining personal hygiene practices, such as cleaning your teeth, taking a bath, and washing your hands. For younger kids, add entertaining games or rewards to make hygiene practices interesting.

Handle Stress: To assist family members in properly handling stress, teach them stress-reduction methods include deep breathing, awareness, and relaxation activities. Promote candid conversation and offer assistance when things are tough.

Set a Good Example: Set a constant example for your family by adopting healthy practices. Since deeds speak louder than words, model positive attitudes and behaviors in your day-to-day activities.

Celebrate Successes: As a family, acknowledge and commemorate accomplishments and significant anniversaries. Acknowledge the work made to create and uphold healthy behaviors, and employ constructive criticism to motivate sustained engagement.

Be Adaptable: Show that you are prepared to modify your habits and routines to fit shifting needs, preferences, and situations. Maintaining long-term devotion to good practices requires flexibility.

You may provide a supportive environment that encourages everyone to make good lifestyle choices and supports general well-being by establishing healthy routines and habits that are customized to your family's requirements and preferences.

As necessary, adapt and adjust

Being flexible and adaptable is essential to keeping your family's routines and habits healthy. Because life is dynamic, things could change and you'll need to modify your strategy. Here's how to modify and refine your tactics as necessary in an efficient manner:

Regularly Evaluate Progress: Allocate some time each month to evaluate the effectiveness of your family's routines and behaviors. Consider your strengths and areas for improvement. Ask family members for their opinions to obtain a variety of viewpoints.

Determine Challenges: Determine any barriers or difficulties that might be making it difficult for your family to maintain routines and good habits. Time restrictions, competing schedules, a lack of drive, or outside pressures are a few examples of this.

Be Willing to Adjust: Have an open mind and be prepared to modify your strategy when necessary. Understand that a family member's wants and preferences may vary, therefore be adaptable in your approach to suit each person's needs and preferences.

Collaborate to Solve Problems: When difficulties emerge, involve your family members in the process of finding solutions. As a team, come up with a list of possible fixes and collaborate to put the modifications that address the root causes into practice.

Modify Expectations and objectives: If you observe that your family is having trouble achieving particular expectations or objectives, think about modifying them to something more reasonable and doable. To encourage advancement, break down more ambitious objectives into smaller, more doable steps.

Adjust Routines: Make necessary adjustments to your family's routines to better fit your present schedules and priorities. This could include changing when you eat, rearranging when you spend time exercising, or adding new activities to your daily or weekly schedule.

Remain Adaptable: Make flexibility and adaptability the cornerstones of your strategy for upholding routines and habits that promote health. Understand that things in life can change at any time, and be ready to modify your plans as necessary.

Communicate Changes: If you make any adjustments to your routines or tactics, let your family members know. To make sure that everyone is in agreement and feels involved in the decision-making process, communication is essential.

Celebrate Progress: Acknowledge all accomplishments and advancements, no matter how slight. Even if your family has faced obstacles along the way, acknowledge the work they have put up and the actions they have done to reach their objectives.

Learn from Experience: Make the most of your past encounters to improve how you approach upholding routines and good behaviors. Make a note of the things that have historically worked well and the things that should be enhanced going forward.

You may establish a framework that will last for the duration of your family's healthy routines and habits by continuing to be flexible and making necessary adjustments to your techniques.

Accept change as a necessary component of the process and never waver in your commitment to your family's welfare.

Promote Responsibility and Progress Monitoring

Promoting accountability and monitoring advancement are useful tactics for keeping your family members inspired and dedicated to their well-being and health objectives. Here's how to put these tactics into practice:

Establish Clear Expectations: Clearly state the objectives and demands for every family member's health and wellbeing. Make sure that everyone is aware of the expectations placed on them and the significance of taking responsibility for reaching these objectives.

Create Accountability Partners: Assign family members to accountable partners who may assist and motivate one another to accomplish their objectives. Accountability partners can encourage one another, hold one another accountable for their activities, and conduct frequent check-ins.

Employ Visual aides: Make charts, calendars, or progress trackers to serve as visual aides for tracking each family member's advancement toward their objectives. Place these visual aids in a prominent area so that everyone can see them, and make sure to update them frequently.

Plan Frequent Check-Ins: Arrange frequent check-in gatherings or conversations to assess advancements, talk about obstacles, and rejoice together as a family. Make the most of these check-ins to offer assistance, solicit feedback, and modify objectives as necessary.

Promote Self-Monitoring: Assist family members in keeping a journal, using applications, or wearing wearable technology to monitor their own development. Self-monitoring gives people control over their health-related behaviors and offers insightful information about their routines and trends.

Celebrate Success: As a family, celebrate successes and milestones to encourage positive behavior and ongoing development.

Acknowledge and commend every family member's endeavors, regardless of their size, and jointly commemorate accomplishments.

Provide Incentives and prizes: Provide incentives and prizes to encourage family members to continue working toward their objectives and staying accountable. Small snacks, special treatment, or enjoyable family activities could all be used as rewards.

Encourage and Support: As family members strive toward their objectives, offer them words of encouragement and support. Encourage others through difficult times and provide support or direction when required.

Lead by Example: Set an example for others to follow by exhibiting a constant dedication to your personal health and well-being objectives. Your family members will be encouraged and inspired to perform similarly by your example.

Think and Adjust: Consider your family's development on a regular basis and assess how well your accountability plans are working. To better meet your family members' wants and preferences, be receptive to their input and modify your strategy as necessary.

You may foster a supportive environment where your family members feel empowered to take charge of their health and well-being and collaborate to achieve their objectives by promoting accountability and monitoring their progress.

Seek Expert Advice and Assistance

Optimizing your family's health and well-being can greatly benefit from professional advice and assistance. The following are some strategies for involving a professional in your family's pursuit of improved health:

Consult Healthcare Providers: To determine the general health of your family and to address any specific conditions or concerns, make regular appointments with pediatricians, family physicians, and specialists. Medical specialists can provide screenings, treatment plans, and individualised recommendations based on the requirements of your family.

See Nutritionists or Dietitians: If you'd want professional advice on meal planning, good eating practices, and your family's nutritional needs, think about scheduling a consultation with one of these professionals. These experts can assist you with creating customized meal plans, taking care of dietary issues, and navigating dietary restrictions or food allergies.

Collaborate with Personal Trainers or Fitness Coaches: Hire personal trainers or fitness coaches to create family-specific workout plans. These experts may offer direction on safe and efficient exercise regimens, appropriate form, and progression, in addition to providing accountability and inspiration.

Attend Counseling or Therapy Sessions: To address mental health difficulties, stress management, marital issues, or behavioral obstacles, seek out counseling or therapy sessions for individual family members or the entire family. Counselors and therapists can provide assistance, coping mechanisms, and methods for enhancing general wellbeing.

Take Part in Parenting Workshops or Support Groups: Attend parenting workshops or support groups to meet other families going through a similar situation and to get advice from professionals in behavior control, child development, and parenting techniques. These groups can provide insightful information, helpful resources, and consoling support.

Investigate Community Resources: Make use of community resources provided by nearby organizations, educational institutions, or healthcare professionals, such as health fairs, workshops, classes, and support groups. These resources frequently offer insightful data as well as chances to network with other families and professionals.

Make Use of Internet Resources: Go to reliable websites, discussion boards, and educational resources offered by reputed businesses, trade associations, and governmental entities. These sites provide a multitude of knowledge on a range of health-related subjects, such as treatment, prevention, and advice for leading a healthy lifestyle.

Examine Telehealth Services: If in-person appointments are not practical or convenient, consider using telehealth services to obtain expert advice and support from a distance. Telehealth appointments are provided by numerous healthcare practitioners for consultations, follow-ups, and continuing assistance.

Take Part in Parenting Classes or Workshops: Sign up for parenting classes or workshops covering subjects like family dynamics, positive discipline, child development, and communication techniques. These courses can offer insightful information and practical tactics for encouraging wholesome family dynamics and constructive conduct.

Keep Yourself Informed and Speak Up for Your Family: When speaking with medical professionals and other professionals, make sure you are aware of the most recent findings, policies, and advice pertaining to health and wellness. You should also speak up for your family's needs and preferences.

You can get access to specialist knowledge, tools, and techniques to assist your family in achieving maximum health and well-being by obtaining professional advice and assistance. Professionals are available to help you along the way, so don't be afraid to ask for help when you need it.

CHAPTER FOUR

Honor accomplishments and maintain momentum

Maintaining commitment and enthusiasm for health and well-being objectives in your family requires acknowledging accomplishments and keeping the momentum going. Here's how to maintain the momentum and celebrate accomplishments:

Celebrate and Honor Accomplishments: Give due recognition to both individual and group accomplishments. Acknowledge accomplishments, goals reached, and strides made toward better routines and habits.

Celebrate Together: Plan unique events, trips, or activities that the whole family will love to commemorate accomplishments. A game day, a picnic in the park, a family movie night, or a healthy culinary competition are a few examples of this.

Establish Rituals or Traditions: Create rituals or traditions to commemorate important anniversaries or triumphs in the field of health and wellbeing. Establish routines that uplift and unite the family, such as a monthly dance party, a quarterly wellness challenge, or a yearly celebration with a health theme.

Reward Efforts: To encourage family members to keep moving forward and to acknowledge their efforts, give them prizes or incentives.

Small pleasures, rights, or worthwhile activities that fit your family's interests and values could all be considered rewards.

Exchange Success Stories: To encourage and uplift one another, family members should exchange success stories and life lessons. Invite family members to talk about their successes, obstacles they've conquered, and life lessons they've discovered.

Consider Your Family's Progress: Give yourself some time to consider how far your family has come in achieving its health and wellbeing objectives. Honor the progress you've made and the favorable adjustments and advancements you've made.

Establish New Objectives: Continue the momentum by establishing fresh objectives and challenges for your family to pursue. Inspire everyone to come up with ideas, establish priorities, and make a commitment to working together to pursue new goals.

Retain Consistency: Even after you've experienced achievement, stick to your healthy routines and behaviors. Maintaining momentum and avoiding relapses into old behaviors require consistency. Maintain your focus on health and wellbeing as a continuous process as opposed to a final goal.

Encourage and support one another as you help family members on their ongoing journeys toward health and well-being. Honor accomplishments, give inspiration when things are tough, and lend a helping hand when required.

Remember to enjoy Every Step: No matter how tiny, never forget to enjoy each accomplishment. Every wise decision and constructive endeavor toward leading a healthier lifestyle should be praised and celebrated.

Your family can develop a resilient, upbeat, and motivated culture by acknowledging and appreciating one other's achievements. Accept every accomplishment as a first step toward a better, healthier future as a team.

CONCLUSION

In summary, making your family's health and well-being a priority is a journey that calls for perseverance, hard work, and a shared resolve to make positive changes. You may empower your family members to make healthier decisions and have more fulfilled lives by putting tactics like encouraging open communication, having clear goals, leading by example, and creating a supportive environment into practice.

This path also requires promoting accountability, obtaining expert advice and assistance, and acknowledging accomplishments. These techniques support the preservation of momentum, tracking of advancement, and motivation throughout time.

Keep in mind that every family is different and that each may need a different approach to better health. On this journey together, embrace adaptability, flexibility, and an attitude of constant growth.

Ultimately, you may build a foundation of health and well-being that enhances the lives of every family member, both now and in the future, by cooperating as a unit, encouraging one another through difficulties, and commemorating victories along the way.

THE END